The Enchanted Garden Sisters

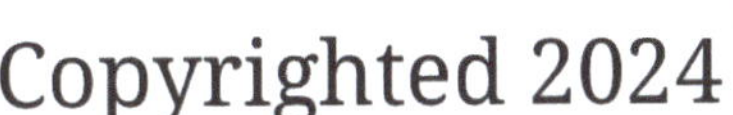

Copyrighted 2024

Author: Chasady Thibodeaux & ChatGpt

Illustrations: Leonardo Ai

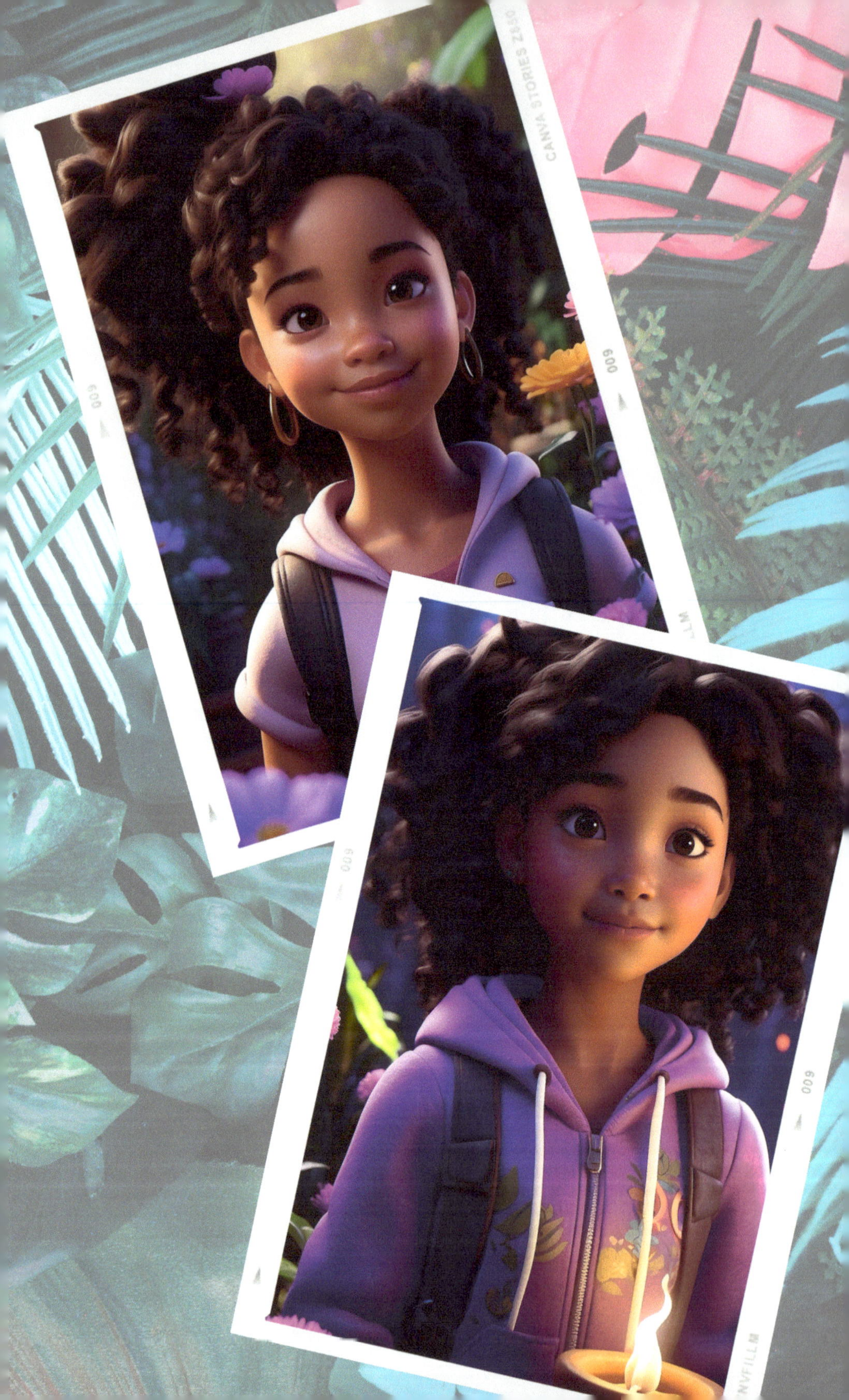

Once upon a time, in the cozy town of Blossomville, lived two sisters named Liyah and Zay. They were always filled with curiosity and a sense of wonder, eager to explore the magic hidden in the world around them.

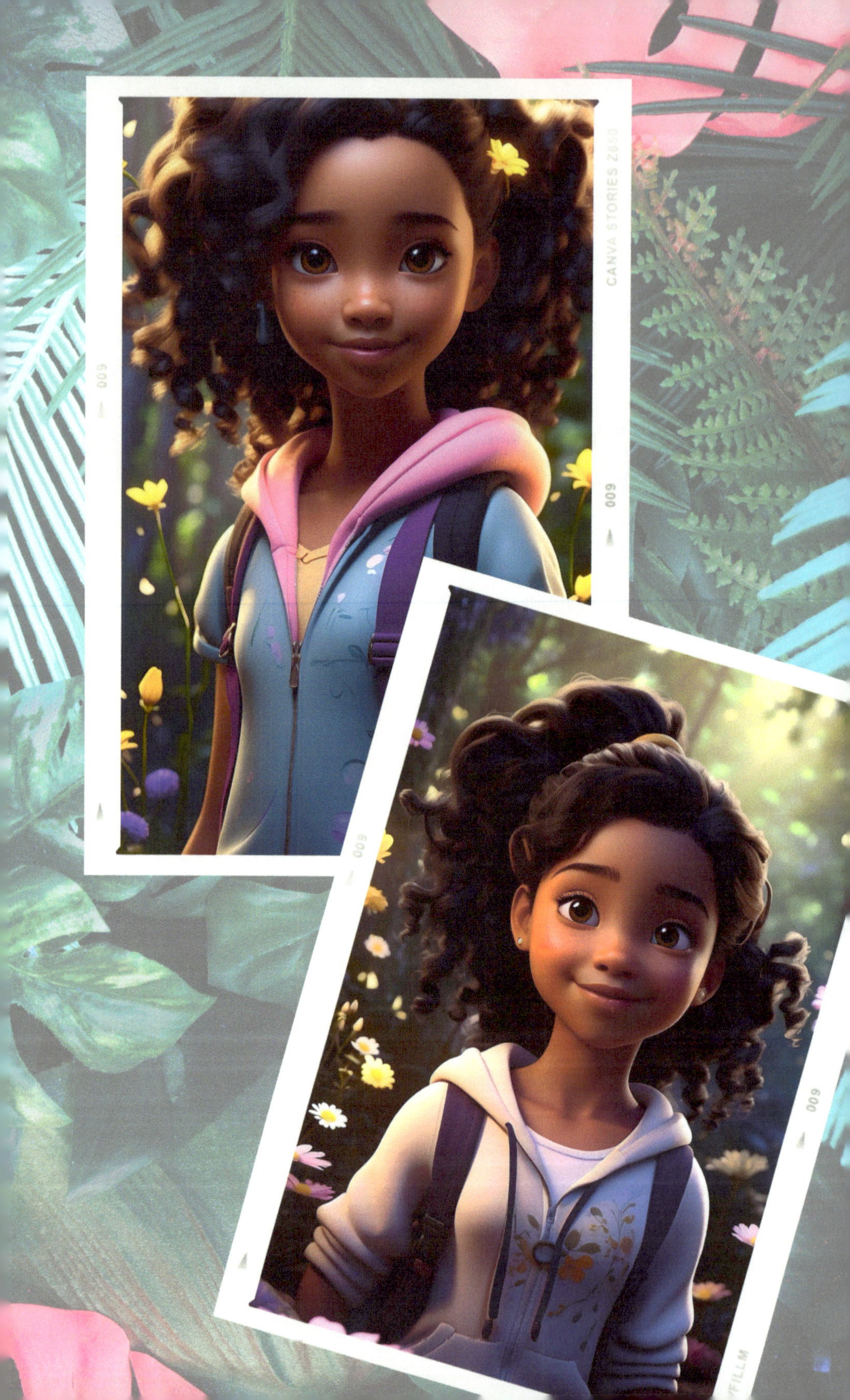

CANVA STORIES Z850
009
009
009
009

One sunny afternoon, as they played in their backyard, a delightful fragrance tickled their noses and beckoned them to discover its source.

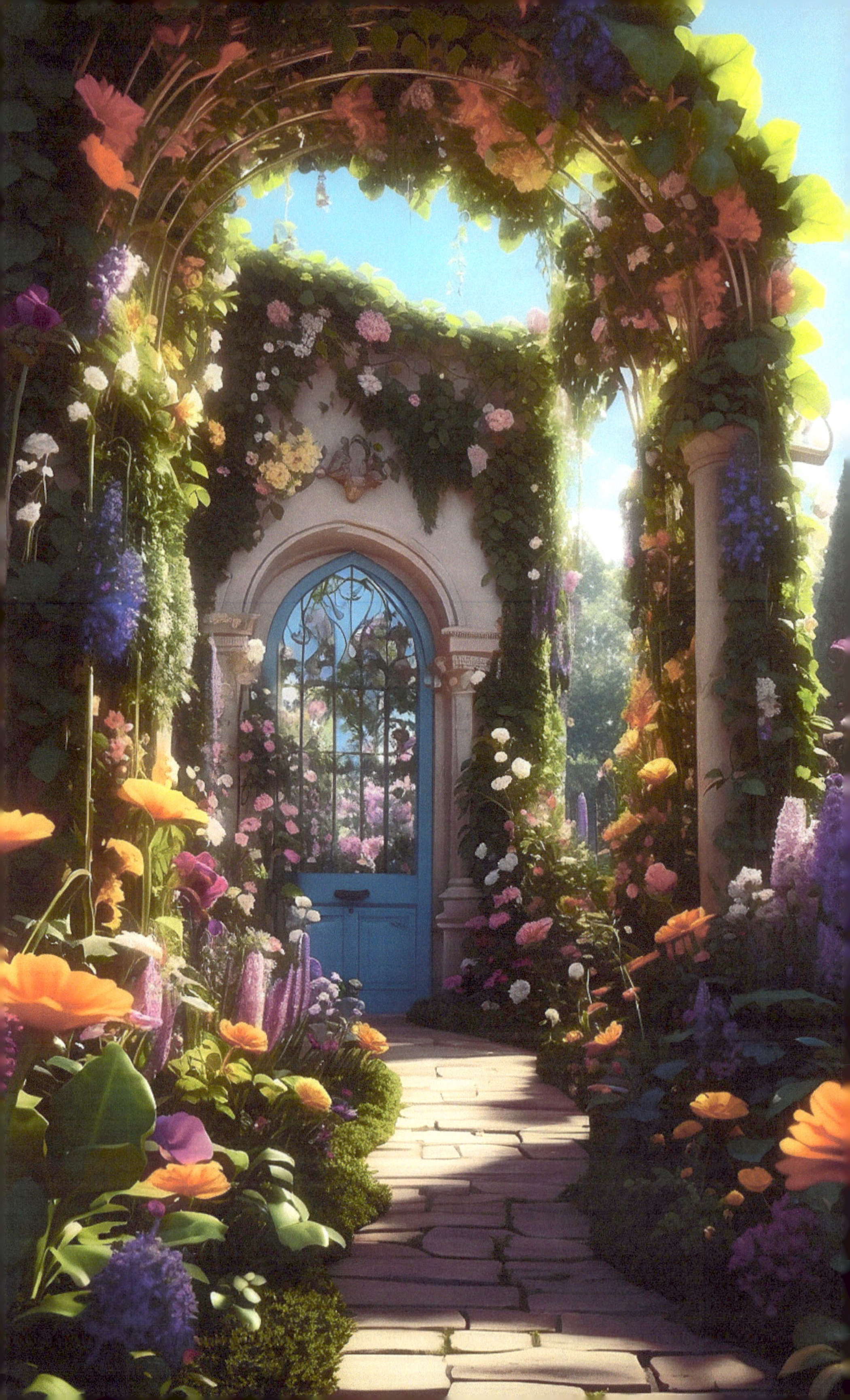

Following the sweet scent, Liyah and Zay found themselves in their mom's enchanting garden, a vibrant oasis filled with blooming flowers and lush greenery.

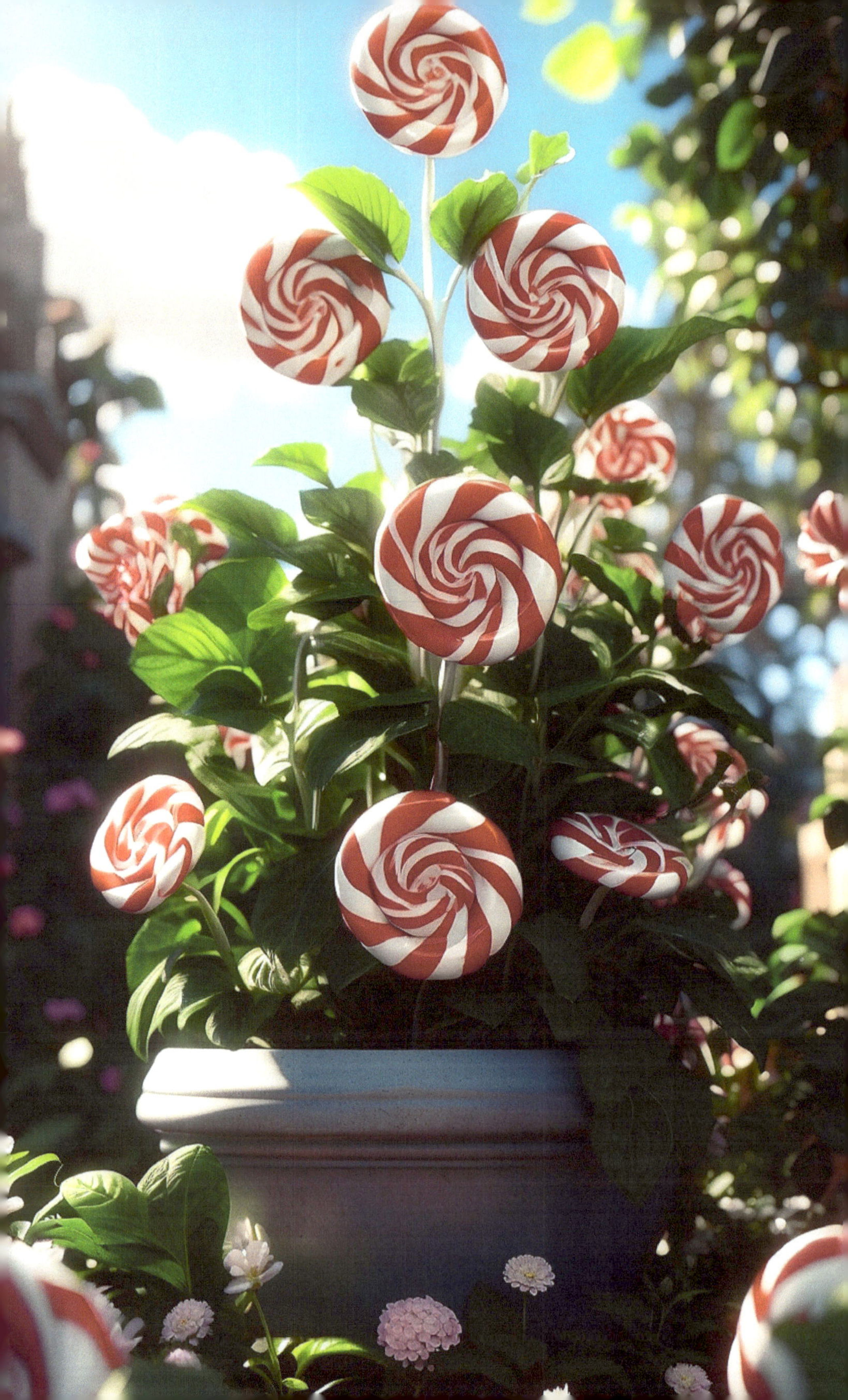

Today, however, held a special surprise; the garden had a secret to share. As the sisters meandered through the rows of colorful blossoms, the scent of peppermint grew stronger.

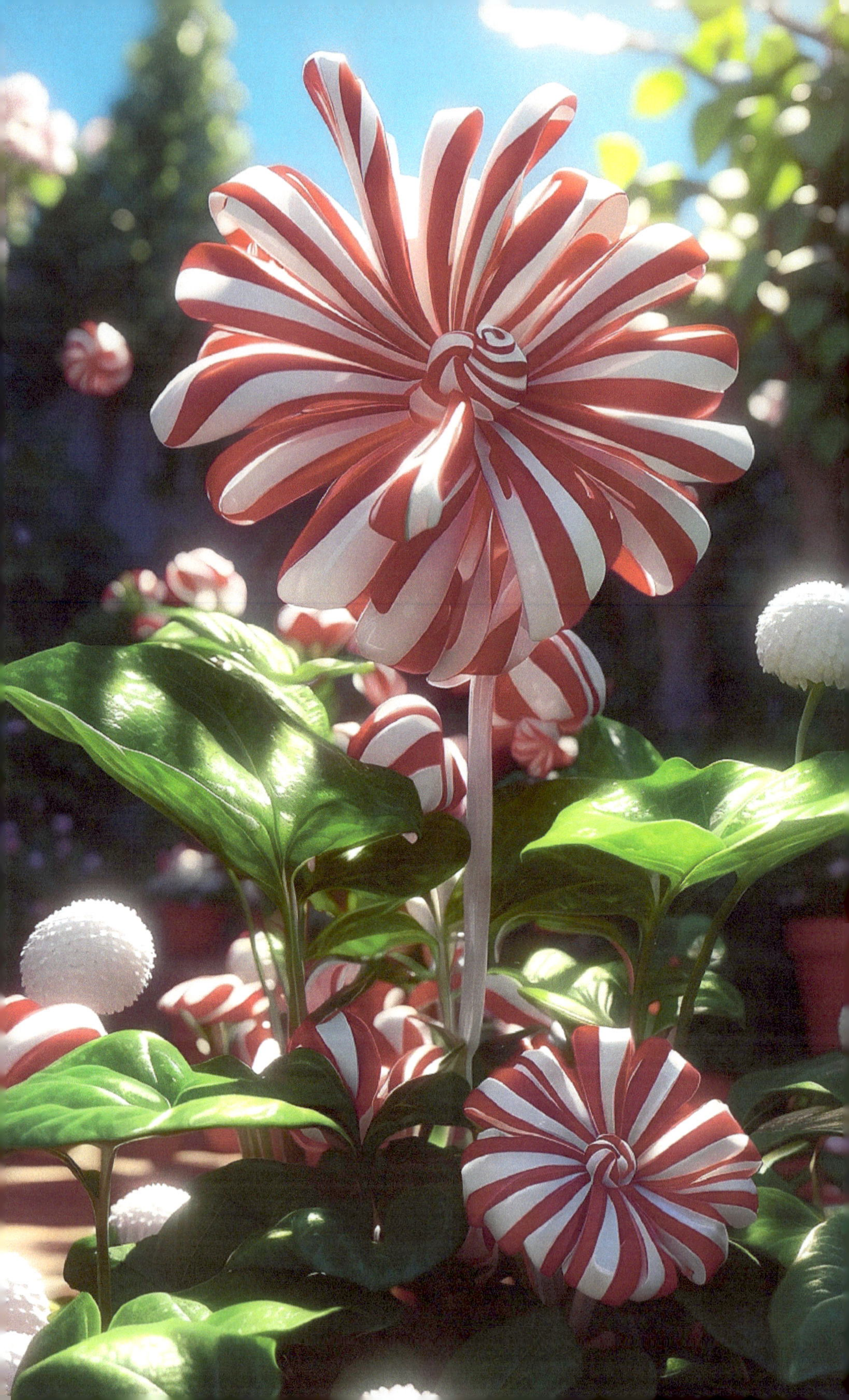

They soon stumbled upon a cluster of small, fragrant peppermint plants. The air was filled with the invigorating aroma, and the sisters couldn't help but giggle with joy.

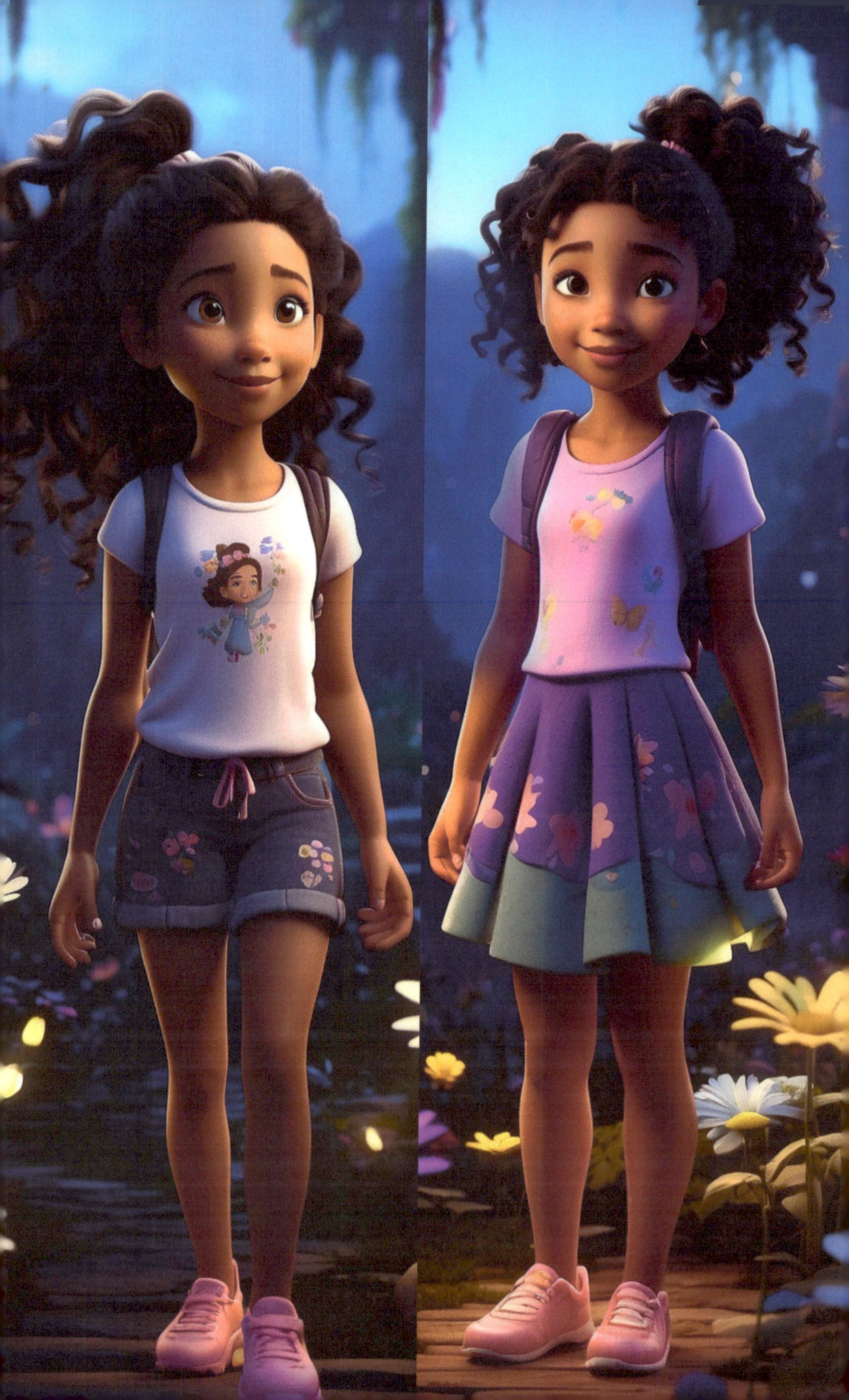

Just as they were

about to pluck a

few peppermint

leaves, a soft,

tinkling voice

chimed in the air,

"Hello, little ones!

What brings you to

my magical

garden?"

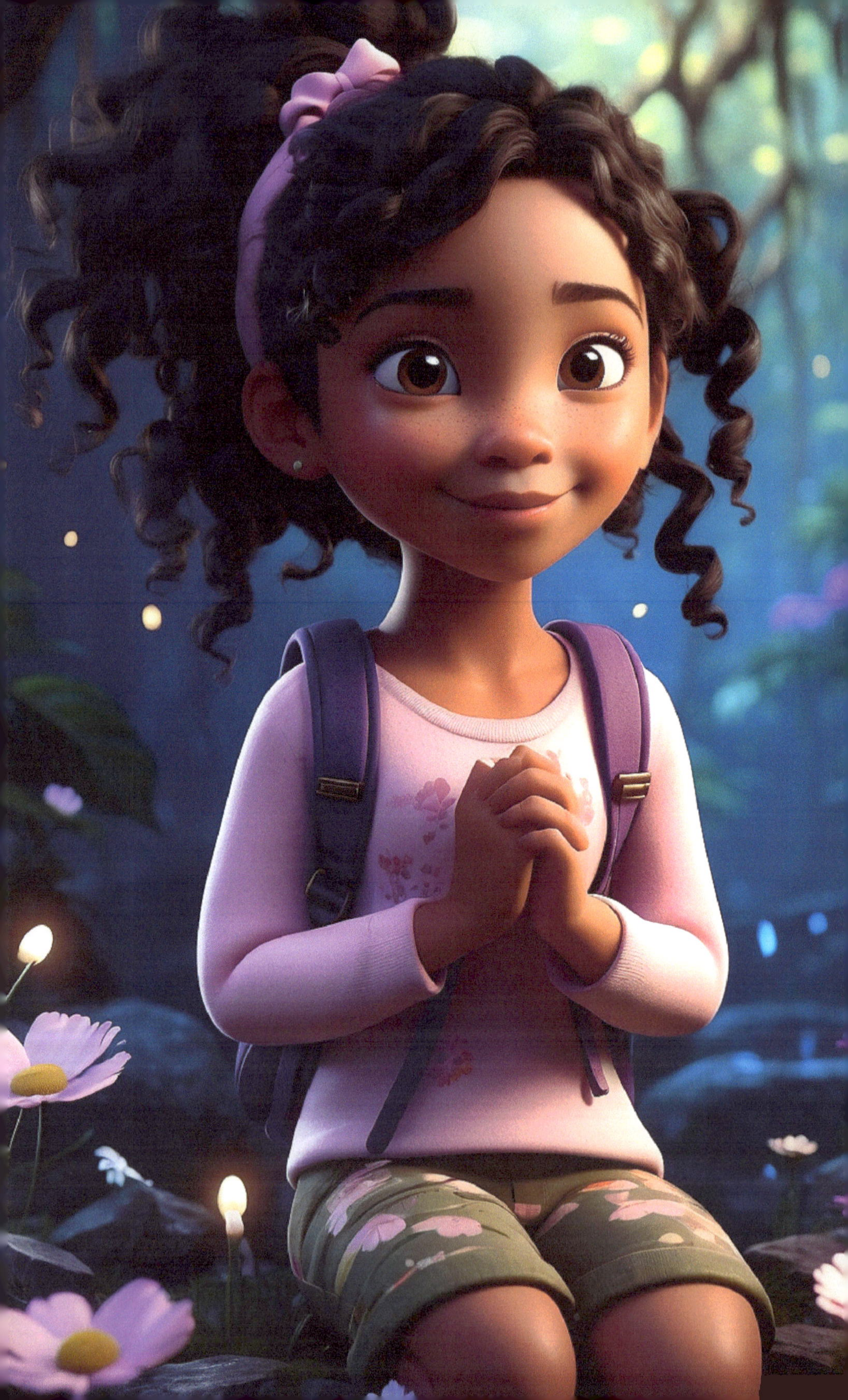

The sisters gasped in amazement as a shimmering figure appeared before them—a fairy with wings adorned in hues of green and petals, her name was Flora.

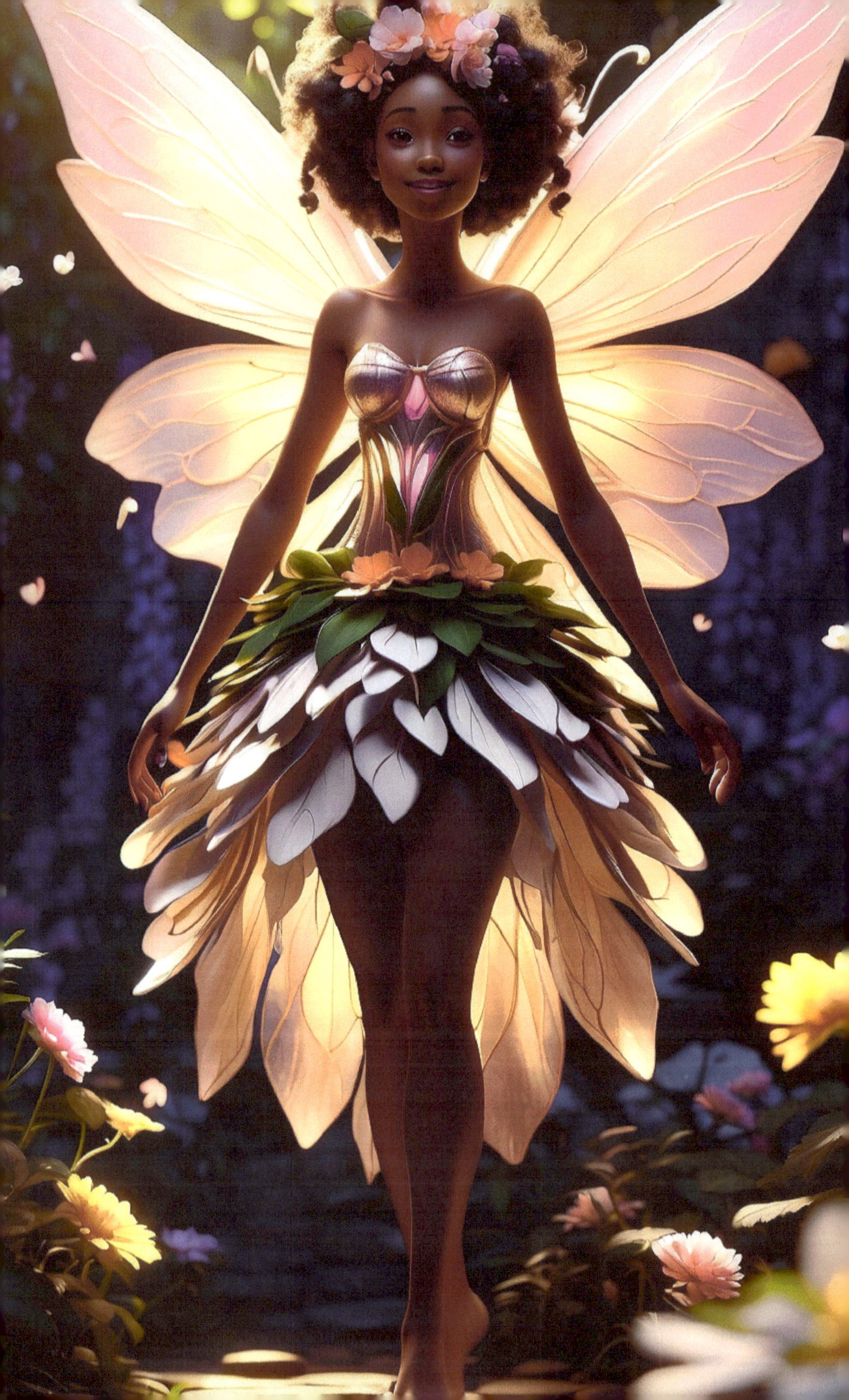

Flora, the garden Fairy, explained, "I am the guardian of these magical plants. I would like to take you to meet the aloe vera plants; it has incredible powers to help us in many ways."

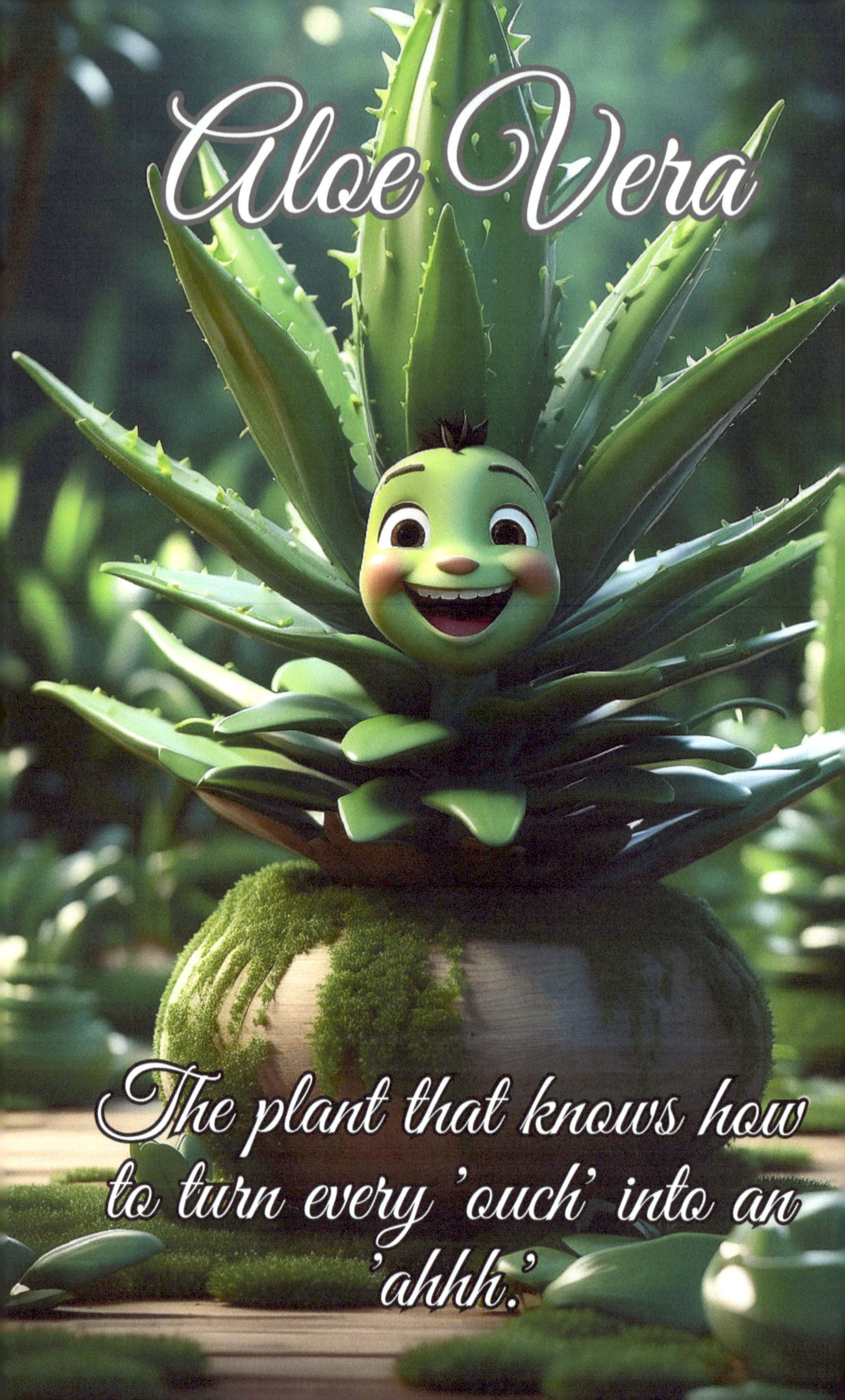

Aloe Vera
The plant that knows how to turn every 'ouch' into an 'ahhh.'

Eager to learn more

about the magical

plants in the garden,

the sisters embarked

on a series of

adventures with

Flora.

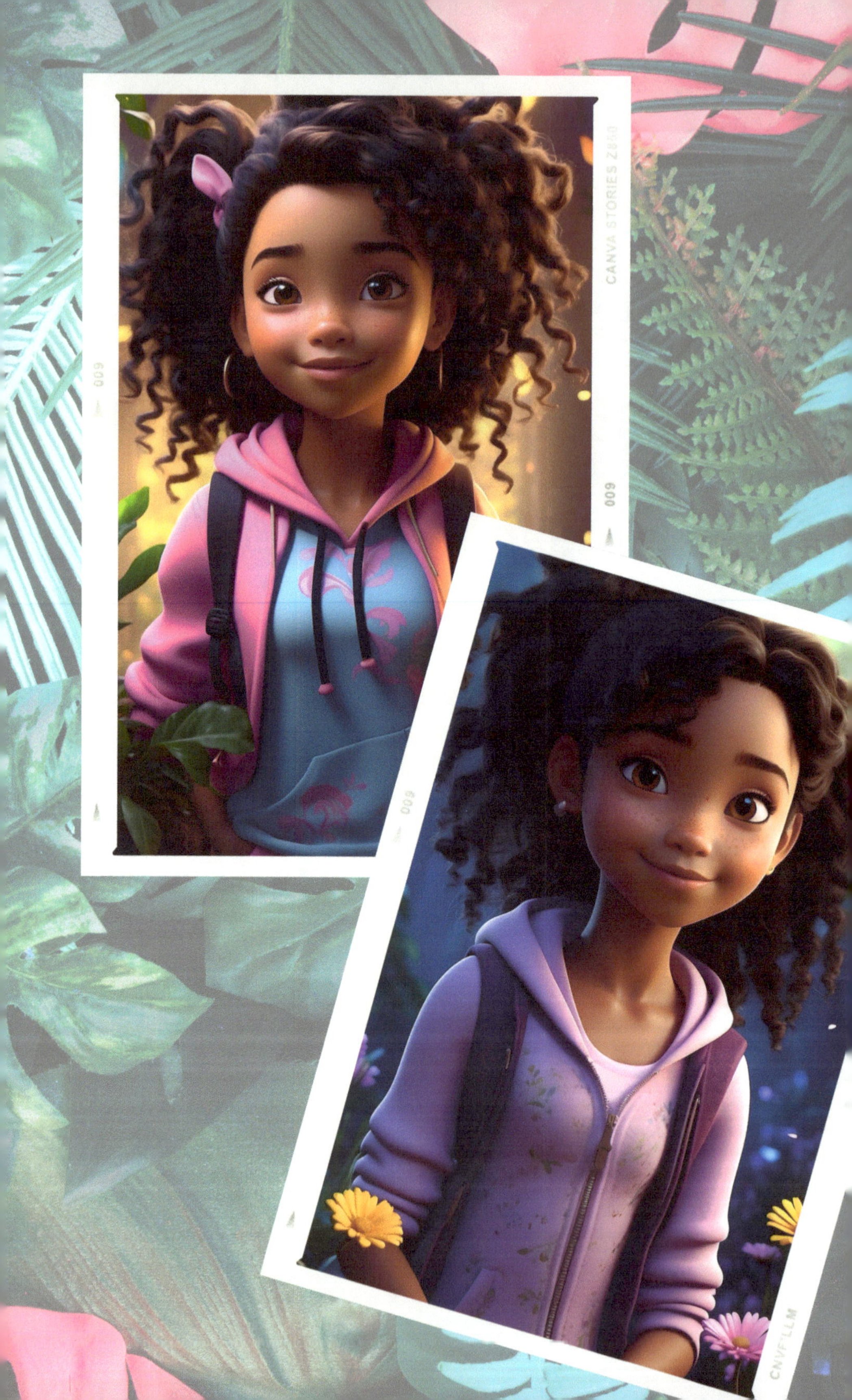

CANVA STORIES Z850
009
009
CNVFILM

They discovered the calming lavender, the healing aloe vera, and the soothing chamomile. Each plant had its unique magic, and the sisters were amazed at the wonders nature had to offer.

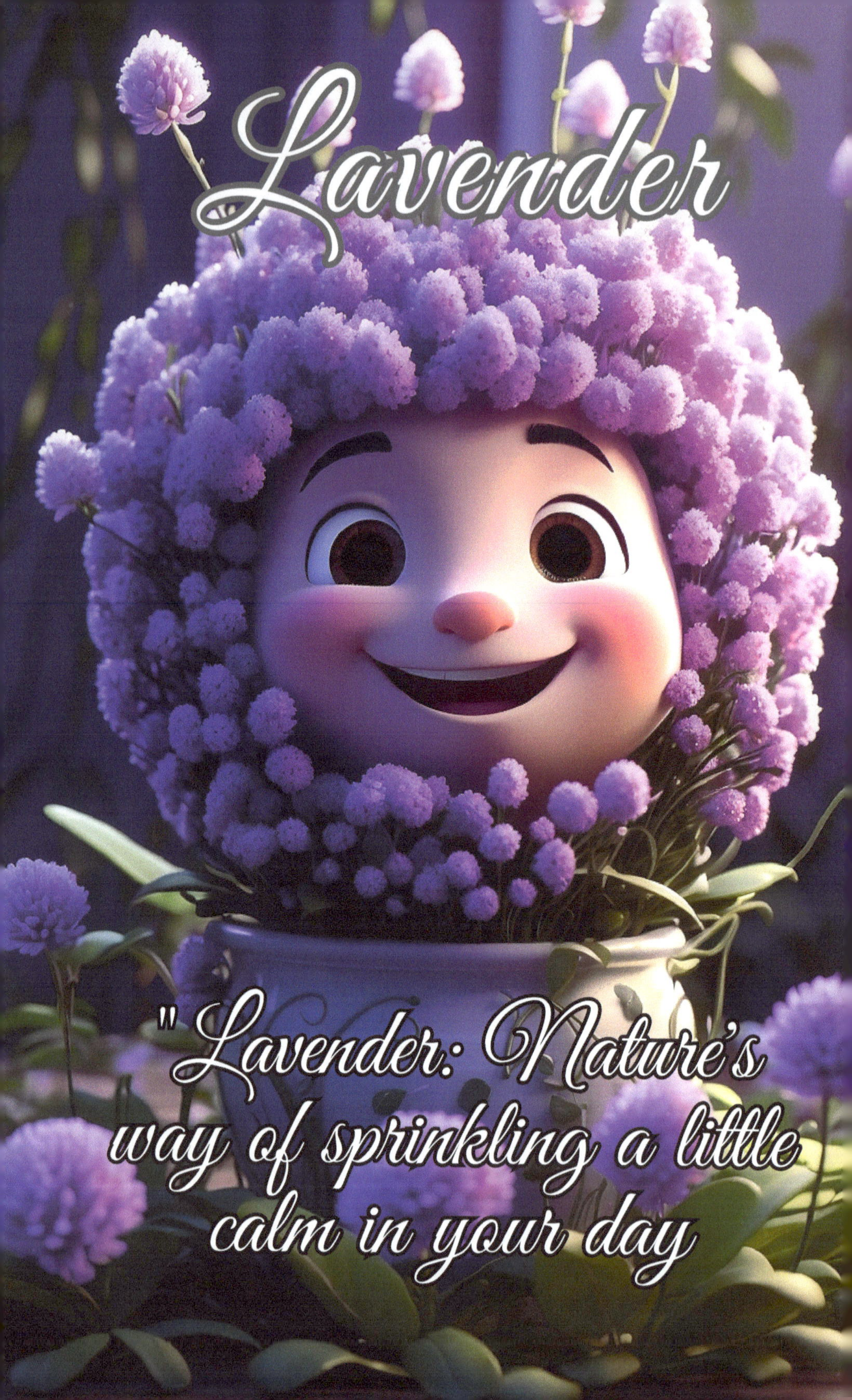

Lavender
"Lavender: Nature's way of sprinkling a little calm in your day

The chamomile plants seemed to come to life, their delicate flowers unfolding into tiny faces with sparkling eyes. "Greetings, dear sisters! I am Cammie, the Chamomile Spirit,"

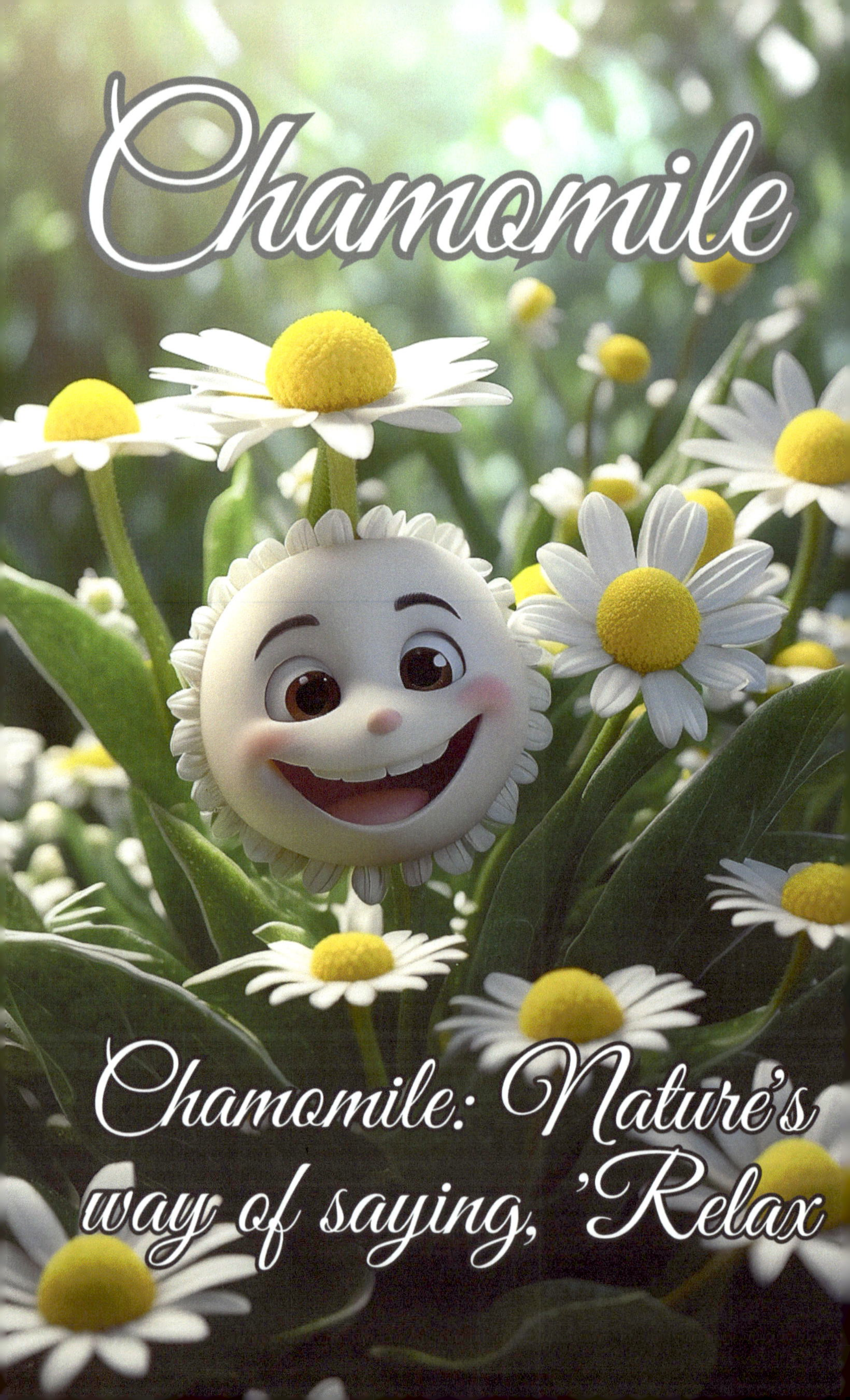

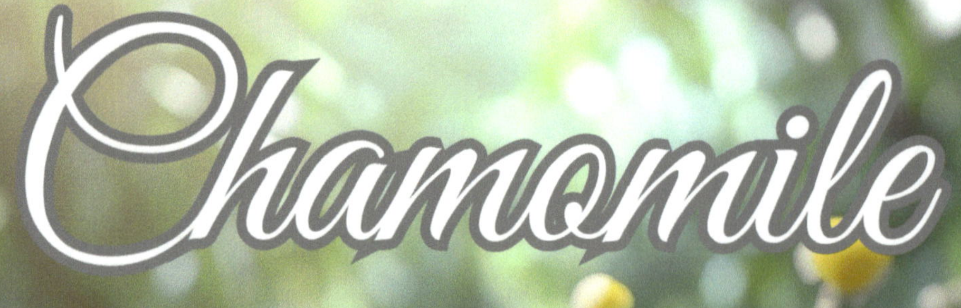

Chamomile

Chamomile: Nature's way of saying, 'Relax

Cammie went on to teach

Liyah and Zay about the

soothing and calming

properties of chamomile.

She explained how

chamomile tea could help

them relax and enjoy

sweet dreams.

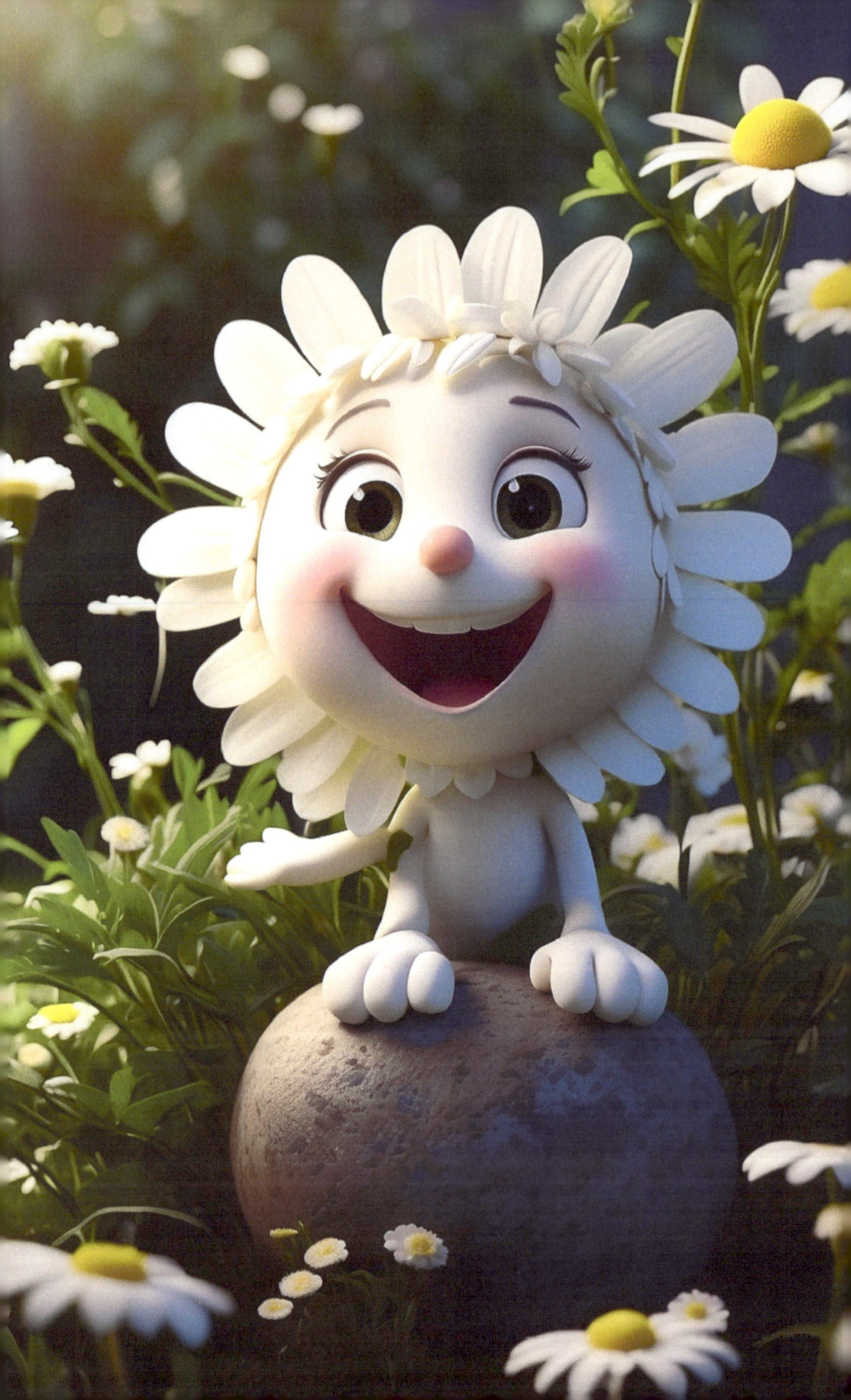

They discovered that
plants were not just
plants; they were
friends with magical
powers waiting to be
explored.

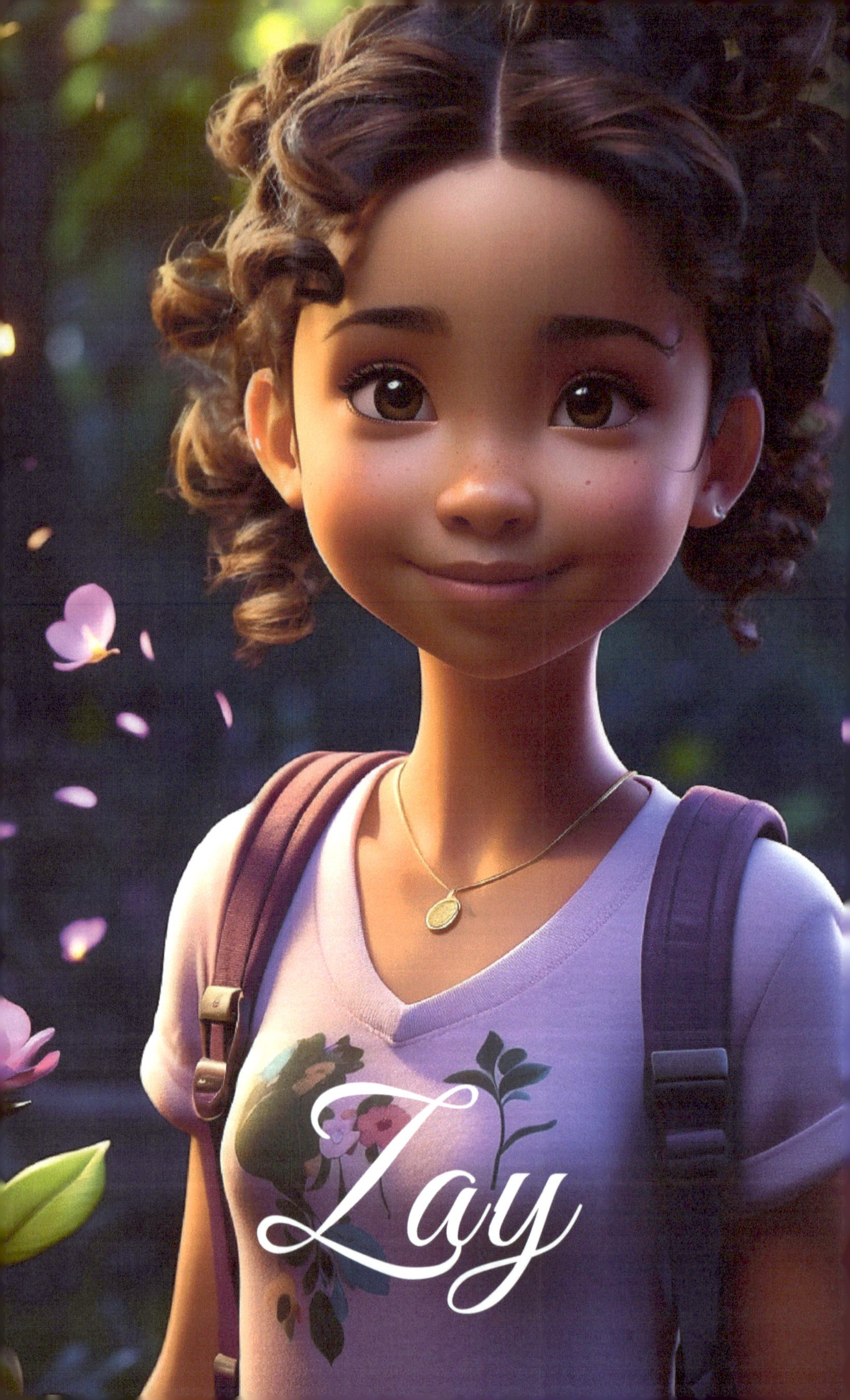
Zay

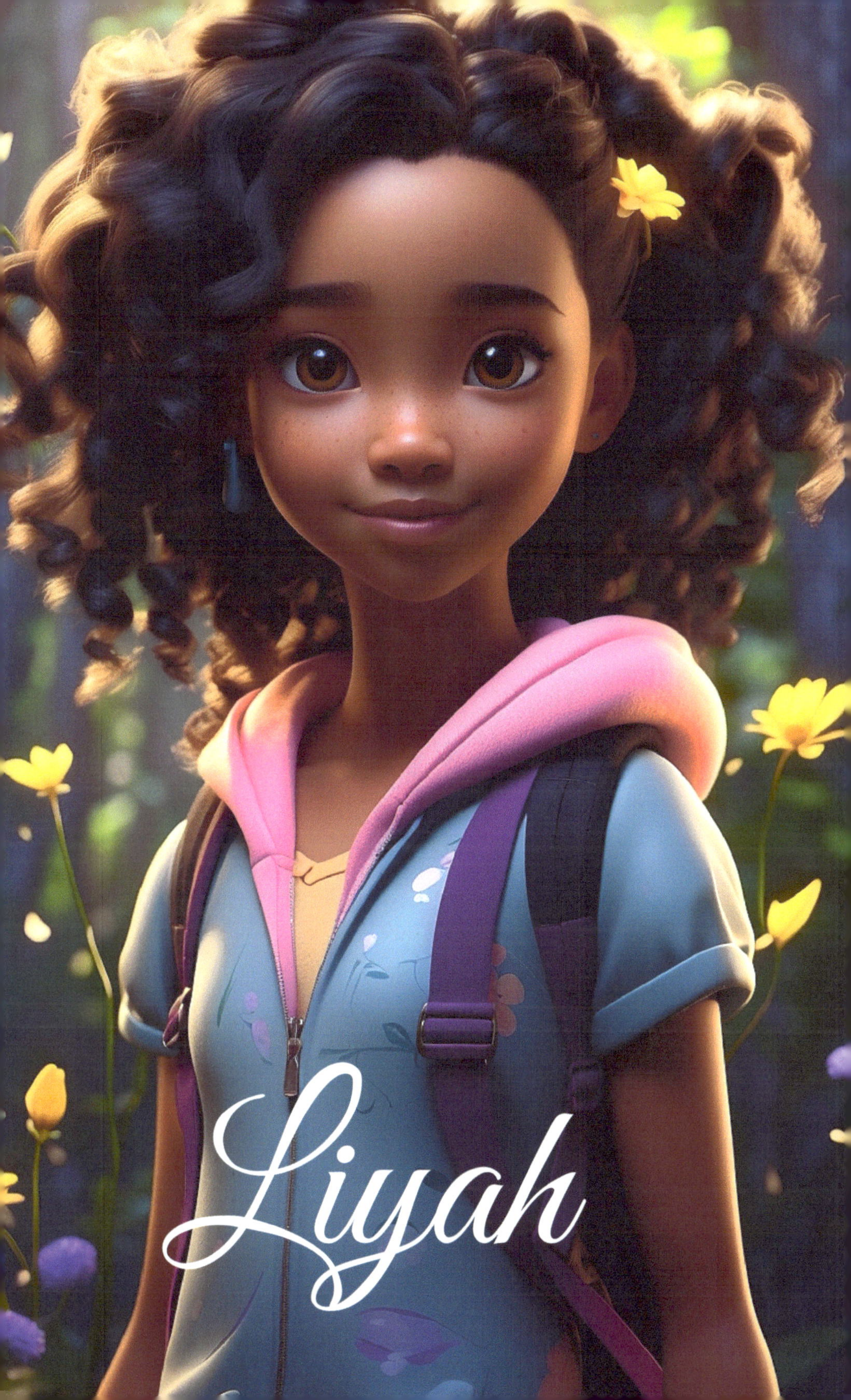
Liyah